I0430045

VARICOSE VEIN NUTRITION FOR NEWLY DIAGNOSED

Optimize Your Diet To Alleviate Symptoms,
Improve Circulation, Reduce Pain, Strengthen
Veins, And Promote Long-Term Wellness

DR. ERIC TRISTAN

CONTENTS

DISCLAIMER

The information provided in this book, is intended for informational purposes only. The content is not intended to be a substitute for professional medical advice, diagnosis, or treatment. Always seek the advice of your physician or other qualified health provider with any questions you may have regarding a medical condition. Never disregard professional medical advice or delay in seeking it because of something you have read in this book.

The author of this book has made reasonable efforts to ensure that the information provided is accurate and up-to-date at the time of publication. However, the author makes no representations or warranties of any kind, express or implied, about the completeness, accuracy, reliability, suitability, or availability of the information contained within these pages.

Any reliance you place on the information provided in this book is strictly at your own risk. The author shall not be liable for any loss, injury, or damage arising from the use of this book or the information contained herein.

The mention or reference to any individuals, products, websites, organizations, or other names within this book does not imply endorsement by the author. The inclusion of such references is solely for informational purposes and does not constitute an endorsement or recommendation.

Furthermore, the author disclaims any association or affiliation with any individuals, products, websites, organizations, or other names mentioned in this book.

It is important to consult with a qualified healthcare professional before making any dietary or lifestyle changes, especially if you have a medical condition. Each individual's health situation is unique, and what works for one person may not work for another.

Again, the information provided in this book is not intended to diagnose, treat, cure, or prevent any disease or health condition. Always seek the advice of a physician or other qualified health provider regarding any medical questions or concerns you may have.

Thank you for your understanding and for taking the necessary precautions when considering the information presented in this book.

ABOUT THIS BOOK

"Varicose Vein Nutrition" is an all-encompassing manual that discusses the vital significance of nutrition in enhancing the well-being of people afflicted with varicose veins. This book commences with a scholarly preface that furnishes readers with a comprehensive synopsis of varicose veins and the ramifications they have on general health. The subsequent section provides an in-depth analysis of varicose veins, including information on their potential complications and underlying causes.

The central theme of this book revolves around the critical significance of nutrition in the management of varicose veins, with particular emphasis on the vital nutrients required to support the veins. The table of contents is extremely well-structured and comprehensive, encompassing various subjects. It even specifies which foods are beneficial for varicose veins and which should be avoided to facilitate effective management. This book delves into the importance of hydration and its influence on the health of varicose veins, illuminating a fundamental element that is frequently disregarded in traditional treatments.

"Varicose Vein Nutrition" addresses lifestyle factors that impact varicose veins in addition to dietary considerations. It also proposes nutritional supplements as a complementary component to a holistic approach. This book presents pragmatic advice on weight management, acknowledging its correlation with varicose veins, and provides nutritional recommendations to enhance circulation. An investigation is conducted into the efficacy of integrating an anti-inflammatory diet into one's regimen as a means of mitigating symptoms and enhancing vascular health.

To aid readers in the practical application of the information, this book provides meal planning recommendations that are specifically designed to promote the health of varicose veins. furthermore, the nutritional guidance offered is complemented by a compilation of delectable recipes that have been meticulously crafted to assist those afflicted with varicose veins. Fundamentally, "Varicose Vein Nutrition" establishes itself as an indispensable resource by providing a comprehensive strategy for the management of varicose veins via lifestyle modifications and informed dietary decisions.

CHAPTER ONE

Introduction

Consisting of vessels that are frequently twisted and distended, varicose veins are a prevalent vascular disorder that impacts millions of individuals across the globe. Although genetics and lifestyle choices are among the many factors that contribute to the development of varicose veins, nutrition is an essential component in both the prevention and management of this condition.

This book aims to examine the complex relationship between nutrition and the health of varicose veins, focusing on fundamental ideas such as the significance of nutrition in vein maintenance and the comprehension of varicose veins.

Comprehension Of Varicose Veins

Before exploring the domain of nutrition, it is crucial to acquire a foundational understanding of varicose veins. The enlargement and twisting of these vessels, which are commonly located in the lower extremities, gives rise to a range of symptoms including pain, edema, and pruritus. Varicose veins manifest due to the weakness or injury of the vein valves, which are vital for the regulation of blood flow. As a consequence of this malfunction, blood accumulates, resulting in the vessels becoming dilated and protruding.

Varicose veins can be attributed to several factors, including advanced age, a familial history of the condition, pregnancy, and extended periods of standing or reclining.

As time passes, the condition has the potential to advance, resulting in physical distress and even complications like venous ulceration. Comprehending the underlying mechanisms of varicose veins is critical to formulating efficacious interventions, such as nutritional methodologies, that mitigate symptoms and avert their exacerbation.

Nutritional Implications For Varicose Vein Health

The influence of nutrition on varicose veins is comparable to that which is crucial for the maintenance of entire vascular health. A balanced diet has the potential to enhance blood circulation, decrease inflammation, and fortify the veins—all of which are critical factors in the management of varicose veins.

Collagen production support is one of the principal nutritional objectives in varicose vein health. As a structural protein, collagen gives the vein walls their rigidity and pliability. It is essential to consume vitamin C-rich foods, as this vitamin is a cofactor in the synthesis of collagen. Strawberries, citrus fruits, and bell peppers are all excellent sources of vitamin C and can be readily implemented into a diet that is kind to the veins.

In addition, it is critical to maintain a healthy weight to alleviate the pressure on the capillaries. Varicose veins can be worsened by the additional pressure that excess body weight places on the lower extremities. A fiber-rich diet, which includes fruits, whole cereals, and legumes, can facilitate weight management and improve digestive health. In addition to aiding in the maintenance of blood volume and preventing dehydration, both of which can cause blood clot formation, adequate hydration is also crucial.

Vital Nutrients For Supporting The Veins

Several nutrients have distinct functions in promoting vein health and alleviating the symptoms associated with varicose veins. Flavonoids, which are present in vegetables and fruits, have been identified as having anti-inflammatory and antioxidant properties. Flavonoids, which are profuse in dark leafy greens, citrus fruits, and berries, have the potential to reduce inflammation and fortify vascular walls.

Omega-3 fatty acids, which are found in abundance in flaxseeds and walnuts, salmon, and mackerel, have been associated with beneficial anti-inflammatory effects for those with varicose veins. By promoting healthy blood circulation and decreasing the risk of blood clot formation, these essential fatty acids facilitate cardiovascular health.

Vitamin E, an additional essential nutrient, promotes the health of blood vessels through its antioxidant properties. To promote vascular health, nuts, seeds, and vegetable oils are excellent sources of vitamin E and can be readily incorporated into a balanced diet.

Varicose vein sufferers may experience advantageous outcomes by incorporating anti-inflammatory nutrients into their diet, in addition to attaining specific nutritional benefits. This entails decreasing the consumption of refined carbohydrates, processed foods, and sugary beverages, as these substances have the potential to exacerbate symptoms and promote inflammation. Conversely, prioritize a dietary regimen abundant in lean proteins, fruits, vegetables, and whole cereals.

In summary, it is critical to comprehend the correlation between varicose veins and nutrition to formulate efficacious approaches for the management and prevention of this prevalent vascular disorder. The implementation of a nutrient-dense, anti-inflammatory diet has the potential to bolster collagen synthesis, fortify capillary walls, and enhance vascular health in general. Furthermore, it is imperative to incorporate adequate hydration and the maintenance of a healthy weight into a comprehensive regimen targeting varicose vein nutrition. By adopting these dietary principles, individuals can proactively alleviate symptoms, promote healthy blood circulation, and sustain vascular health over an extended period.

Incorporating Foods Into A Varicose Vein Diet

A prevalent medical condition, varicose veins manifest as vein enlargement and entanglement, frequently inducing physical discomfort and pain. Diverse factors, including lifestyle and heredity, contribute to the development of varicose veins; however, nutrition is the most important in preventing and managing these conditions. By promoting vascular health and alleviating symptoms associated with this condition, a balanced diet can be of assistance.

1. Consuming foods that are abundant in fiber is critical for the maintenance of healthy blood vessels. Constipation is prevented by fiber, which may contribute to elevated vein pressure. Vegetables, fruits, whole cereals, and legumes are all rich in fiber. Furthermore, by aiding in weight management, these foods reduce the risk of obesity, a well-established risk factor for varicose veins.

2. Foods High in Antioxidants: Antioxidants are crucial for preventing oxidative stress in the blood vessels. Nuts, berries, citrus fruits, and dark verdant vegetables are all excellent sources of antioxidants, including flavonoids and vitamin C. These compounds promote overall vascular health by fortifying capillary walls.

3. Omega-3 Fatty Acids: Individuals afflicted with varicose veins may benefit from the anti-inflammatory properties of omega-3 fatty acids. Fatty fish (including salmon, mackerel, and trout), walnuts, and flaxseeds are all excellent sources of these lipids that are beneficial to the heart. By aiding in the reduction of inflammation and enhancement of blood circulation, omega-3 fatty acids promote vein health.

4. Vitamin E-Rich Foods: Vitamin E is recognized for its potential to promote blood vessel health and its antioxidant properties. Vitamin E-rich foods include almonds, sunflower seeds, asparagus, spinach, and sunflower seeds. These can aid in the maintenance of blood vessel integrity and decrease the likelihood of developing varicose veins.

5. Magnesium is an indispensable mineral for the proper functioning of muscles and nerves, as well as for the maintenance of healthy blood vessels. Whole grains, legumes, leafy vegetables, and seeds are all excellent sources of magnesium.

Magnesium consumption in sufficient quantities promotes healthy arteries and could potentially mitigate the severity of varicose veins.

6. Foods Rich in Potassium: Potassium aids in the regulation of bodily fluid balance, thereby mitigating the likelihood of fluid retention and leg edema—a prevalent manifestation linked to varicose veins. Potassium-rich foods such as bananas, citrus, potatoes, and tomatoes may contribute to the maintenance of cardiovascular health.

CHAPTER TWO

Foods To Avoid For The Management Of Varicose Veins

While specific nutrients are beneficial for vascular health, others may worsen the symptoms of varicose veins. Dietary management through the avoidance of specific foods has the potential to enhance vein health and mitigate the discomfort commonly associated with varicose veins.

1. Consuming foods high in sodium can result in water retention and edema, which in turn elevates the pressure on the vessels. Soups in cans, processed foods, and savory treats are frequent sources of sodium. By restricting sodium consumption, one can effectively regulate fluid retention and alleviate the burden on blood vessels.

2. Carbohydrates and Refined Sugars: Two risk factors for varicose veins are inflammation and weight gain, both of which are influenced by refined sugars and carbohydrates.

It is advisable to restrict the consumption of sweetened treats, white bread, and pastries. By substituting whole grains and complex carbohydrates for other foods, one can aid in weight maintenance and inflammation reduction.

3. Elevated intake of foods that are rich in saturated fats and trans fats has been associated with the development of arterial rigidity and inflammation. By limiting the intake of fried foods, processed munchies, and fatty portions of meat, individuals can enhance their cardiovascular health in general, which encompasses the prevention and treatment of varicose veins.

4. Both alcohol and caffeine have the potential to cause dehydration, which could exacerbate the symptoms associated with varicose veins. In addition, these substances have the potential to cause vasodilation, which may elevate the susceptibility to venous insufficiency. A recommendation is to exercise moderation when it comes to consuming

alcoholic beverages, coffee, and tea for those who are managing varicose veins.

5. Although not classified as a food item, high-heeled shoes have the potential to promote the formation and worsening of varicose veins. Extended periods spent in high heels may hinder adequate blood circulation in the lower extremities. Choosing low-heeled, comfortable footwear improves blood circulation and relieves pressure on the capillaries.

Hydration And The Health Of Varicose Veins

Adequate hydration is an essential component in the management of varicose veins and is fundamental to overall health. Adequate hydration is essential for maintaining healthy blood circulation, preventing thrombosis, and decreasing the likelihood of thrombus formation. The following are critical hydration recommendations for those who have varicose veins:

1.   Water   Consumption: Sufficient   water consumption is critical for sustaining optimal blood viscosity and facilitating optimal blood circulation. Although eight 8-ounce containers of water per day is a recommended minimum, it is important to note that individual hydration requirements may differ. By preventing blood from accumulating in the vessels, adequate hydration decreases the likelihood of developing varicose vein symptoms.

2. Herbal teas, including chamomile and ginger tea, have the potential to aid in hydration while avoiding the diuretic properties typically associated with caffeinated beverages. Additionally, individuals with varicose veins may benefit from the anti-inflammatory properties of these beverages.

3. Restricting Caffeine and Alcohol Consumption: The consumption of caffeine and alcohol may exacerbate symptoms of varicose veins by contributing to dehydration. Although it is generally permissible to consume in moderation, an inordinate amount should be prevented. Choosing water and

botanical infusions as one's primary beverage options facilitates improved hydration.

4. Incorporating fruits and vegetables that possess a substantial water content, including watermelon, cucumber, and celery, into one's diet may enhance overall hydration. In addition to providing hydration, these foods also contain vital nutrients that promote vascular health.

5. Although not directly associated with hydration, the utilization of compression stockings may assist in the management of varicose veins. By promoting blood circulation through the application of pressure to the legs, these garments alleviate discomfort and edema. Having a hydrated epidermis facilitates the comfortable donning of compression stockings.

In summary, the effective management of varicose veins requires the consumption of a balanced diet that is abundant in vital vitamins and minerals, fiber, antioxidants, and omega-3 fatty acids.

In addition to remaining hydrated, avoiding foods high in sodium, sugar, and fat contributes to overall vascular health. The management and prevention of varicose veins can be substantially enhanced by incorporating lifestyle modifications, including consistent exercise and the use of compression stockings, in addition to the aforementioned dietary measures. Always seek the personalized guidance of a healthcare professional regarding your particular health condition and requirements.

An Exhaustive Guide To Varicose Vein Nutrition

Varicose veins are a prevalent vascular disorder characterized by the enlargement and twisting of blood vessels; they typically affect the lower extremities. Although age and genetics are major contributors to the development of varicose veins, their severity and progression can also be affected by lifestyle and dietary decisions. This guide will examine the influence of nutrition on varicose veins, with a specific emphasis on weight management, nutritional supplements, anti-inflammatory regimens, and lifestyle factors.

Aspects Of Lifestyle That Influence Varicose Veins

The direction of one's lifestyle significantly influences the progression and onset of varicose veins. Insufficient physical activity, protracted periods of inactivity (standing or reclining), and sedentary behavior can all contribute to compromised blood circulation, resulting in elevated vein pressure. To alleviate these factors, inhabitants may integrate uncomplicated modifications into their daily regimen.

Consistent physical activity is essential for enhancing blood circulation. Participating in physical exercises such as walking, swimming, or cycling contributes to the fortification of the calf muscles, which are crucial for the return of circulation to the heart. In addition, during the course of the day, stretching and moving pauses can help prevent blood from accumulating in the legs.

Additionally, maintaining a healthy weight is critical for the prevention and treatment of varicose veins. A surplus of body weight exerts additional strain on the vessels, thereby impeding the correct circulation of blood. In addition to aiding in weight management, consistent exercise and the adoption of a well-balanced diet can assist in the prevention of varicose veins.

Additionally, compression stockings can deliver vein support and aid in symptom relief. By exerting mild compression on the lower extremities, these stockings promote circulation and inhibit the accumulation of blood.

Despite being frequently neglected, hydration is vital for vascular health. Adequate water consumption aids in the maintenance of blood volume and promotes cardiovascular health. Blood that is too thin can result from dehydration, which can increase the risk of blood clotting and worsen the symptoms of varicose veins.

CHAPTER THREE

Supplementary Nutrition For Varicose Veins

Diverticone sufferers may also find it advantageous to include particular nutritional supplements in their dietary regimen, in conjunction with making adjustments to their way of life. Specific minerals and micronutrients promote vascular health and may aid in symptom management.

1. Vitamin C is indispensable for the synthesis of collagen, a substance that is critical for the integrity and pliability of blood vessels. By incorporating vitamin C-rich foods into one's diet, such as bell peppers, citrus fruits, and strawberries, vascular health can be improved.

2. Vitamin E: Due to its antioxidant properties, vitamin E aids in the protection of blood vessel lining cells. Leafy green vegetables, nuts, and seeds are all excellent sources of vitamin E.

3. Flavonoids, which are derived from plants, possess antioxidant and anti-inflammatory properties that may promote vascular health. Flavonoid-rich foods consist of green tea, berries, citrus fruits, and scallions.

4.Omega-3 fatty acids, which are present in walnuts, fatty salmon, and flaxseeds, possess anti-inflammatory characteristics that potentially alleviate symptoms related to varicose veins.

5. Horse Chestnut Seed Extract: The potential of this herbal supplement to increase blood flow and decrease leg edema has been investigated. Nevertheless, it is imperative to seek the advice of a healthcare professional before integrating any botanical supplements into one's daily regimen.

Although these supplements may provide some alleviation, acquiring nutrients predominantly through a variegated and well-balanced diet is of utmost importance. It is advisable to seek guidance from a healthcare professional before commencing any supplementation regimen.

A Diet Low In Inflammation To Treat Varicose Veins

An element that contributes to the development and progression of varicose veins is inflammation. A diet rich in anti-inflammatory foods can aid in inflammation management and improve vascular health overall.

1. Fruits and Vegetables: Anti-inflammatory antioxidants are abundant in vibrant fruits and vegetables. Kale, berries, cherries, and chard are all outstanding options.

2. Fatty Fish Salmon, mackerel, and sardines are examples of cold-water fish that are rich in omega-3 fatty acids, which possess anti-inflammatory properties.

3. Choosing whole grains over refined grains is beneficial for the cardiovascular system as they contain fiber and vital nutrients.

4. Nuts and Seeds: Almonds, walnuts, and flaxseeds contain anti-inflammatory compounds and healthful lipids.

5. Herbs and spices possess considerable anti-inflammatory properties and are readily incorporateable into a wide range of dishes, including turmeric, ginger, and garlic.

A lifestyle that is low in red meat, industrial foods, and caffeinated beverages can also be reduced to promote anti-inflammatory health.

Management Of Body Weight And Varicose Veins

It is essential to maintain a healthy weight to prevent and manage varicose veins. An accumulation of body fat places an additional burden on the vascular system and impairs blood circulation by putting pressure on the vessels.

1. A well-balanced diet, consisting primarily of whole cereals, fruits, vegetables, and lean proteins, has the potential to positively impact weight

management. It is essential to ration portions and prevent excessive caloric consumption.

2. Consistent Physical Activity: Maintaining a routine schedule for physical activity is critical for effectively managing body weight and enhancing circulation. Engaging in physical activities such as cycling, walking, and swimming can strengthen the muscles that support healthy venous function and aid in weight loss.

3. Hydration: Adequate water consumption promotes overall health and may assist with weight management. Occasionally, the body may misinterpret thirst for appetite, resulting in the consumption of extra calories.

4. Crash diets, which involve rapid weight loss, should be avoided due to their potential adverse effects on vascular health. Adopting sustainable lifestyle modifications that facilitate incremental and healthful weight loss is of utmost importance.

5. Seeking Advice from Healthcare Professionals: When considering weight management for varicose veins, individuals should seek guidance from healthcare professionals, including dietitians and physicians. They can offer customized guidance and assistance for specific health conditions and requirements.

In summary, a comprehensive strategy for varicose vein nutrition encompasses the integration of specific nutritional supplements, adherence to an anti-inflammatory diet, and proficient weight management, all of which contribute to a healthy lifestyle. The integration of these approaches can enhance the prevention and control of varicose veins, thereby fostering the general health and welfare of the vascular system. When dealing with any matter about health, it is imperative to seek personalized advice and direction from healthcare professionals.

CHAPTER FOUR

Varicose Vein Nutrition: Enhancing Vein Health Through Nutrient Intake

Many people find varicose veins, which are veins that frequently enlarge contort, and manifest on the legs, to be a source of distress and concern. Although numerous medical interventions are accessible, nutrition remains an essential factor in the management and prevention of varicose veins. By promoting enhanced circulation, a balanced diet can decrease the risk of developing these unsightly and occasionally excruciating veins.

Suggestions For Optimising Circulation Via Dietary Means:

1. Flavonoids, which are present in an abundance of fruits and vegetables, are compounds that have been associated with enhanced vascular health. Flavonoids are abundant in leafy vegetables, citrus fruits, cherries, and scallions. By fortifying blood vessels and increasing blood flow, these compounds can help reduce the risk of varicose veins.

2. Expanding Fiber Consumption: Adhering to a diet rich in fiber not only confers advantages for digestive health but also contributes to the promotion of cardiovascular wellness. Vegetables, whole cereals, and legumes have the potential to alleviate capillary pressure, promote circulation, and prevent constipation.

3. Select Omega-3 Fatty Acids: Omega-3 fatty acids, which are present in chia seeds, mackerel, salmon, and fatty fish, possess anti-inflammatory attributes that potentially mitigate symptoms linked to varicose veins. By incorporating these foods into one's dietary regimen, one may potentially enhance blood circulation and mitigate inflammation.

4. Maintaining proper hydration is of utmost importance as vein-related complications can be significantly worsened by dehydration. Water aids in the regulation of blood volume, thereby inhibiting the accumulation of blood that would otherwise strain the vasculature. Consistently consume

sufficient water throughout the day to maintain optimal vascular health.

5. Restrict Sodium Consumption: An overabundance of sodium can result in water retention, which in turn elevates blood vessel pressure. Incorporating less sodium into one's diet can aid in fluid balance management and reduce the likelihood of varicose vein-related complications such as inflammation and edema.

Planning Meals To Promote Varicose Vein Health

By devising a meticulously planned meal regimen, one can effectively guarantee that their body is supplied with the appropriate nutrients necessary to promote vein health.

1. For breakfast, consume a serving of oatmeal that has been seasoned with chia seeds and fruit. In contrast to oats, which contain soluble fiber, berries are rich in flavonoids. Supplemented with omega-3 fatty acids are chia seeds.

2. Salad vegetables, tomatoes, cucumbers, and lean protein such as tofu or grilled chicken constitute a nutritious lunch. In addition to supplying vital vitamins and minerals, the lean protein in these vegetables promotes muscle health.

3. Snacks: Indulge in hazelnuts or almonds, which are excellent sources of omega-3 fatty acids. Greek yogurt accompanied by fresh fruit and a drizzle of honey can also serve as a scrumptious and nourishing substitute.

4. Incorporate a portion of oily fish, such as trout or salmon, into the dinner menu, accompanied by quinoa or brown rice and an assortment of vibrant vegetables. This meal is rich in antioxidants, fiber, and omega-3 fatty acids, all of which promote cardiovascular health.

Recipes For Supporting Varicose Veins

1. Blend one cup of mixed berries (strawberries, blueberries, and raspberries), one banana, one tablespoon of chia seeds, and one cup of low-fat

yogurt to make a berry smoothie. This smoothie is an omega-3 and flavonoid powerhouse, in addition to being incredibly tasty.

2. Salmon fillets for a grilled salmon salad should be marinated in olive oil, lemon juice, and seasonings. Serve the grilled chicken over a mound of mixed greens, cucumbers, and cherry tomatoes. Grill until thoroughly cooked. Utilize a vinaigrette composed of balsamic vinegar and olive oil to drizzle.

3. To prepare quinoa and vegetable stir-fry, follow the cooking instructions on the package. Stir-fry snap peas, bell peppers, and broccoli in a pan with garlic and ginger. Complement the entrée with cooked quinoa and a small amount of low-sodium soy sauce.

4. Chia Seed Pudding: Incorporate chia seeds, almond milk, vanilla extract, and a trace amount of honey. Allow it to rest overnight in the refrigerator. Serve garnished with freshly harvested fruit for a delectable and healthful nibble or dessert.

In summary, adopting a comprehensive approach to varicose vein nutrition has the potential to substantially enhance vein health. By integrating the following suggestions and recipes into your daily regimen, you can promote enhanced circulation and mitigate the likelihood of varicose vein development or exacerbation. Bear in mind that maintaining a nutrient-dense and balanced diet has numerous positive effects, not only on vascular health but also on your overall well-being.

Conclusion

In summary, nutrition serves as an integral component in the management of varicose veins, providing a comprehensive strategy to promote vascular well-being. A diet abundant in foods that arc high in fiber facilitates weight maintenance, thereby mitigating the likelihood of complications associated with obesity that may worsen vascular problems. Additionally, the consumption of fatty salmon, berries, and leafy vegetables, which contain anti-inflammatory properties, may aid in the reduction of inflammation linked to varicose veins.

Vitamin C and flavonoids are essential nutrients that play a role in the synthesis of collagen and fortify the walls of blood vessels, thereby potentially impeding additional harm. Moreover, by preventing oxidative stress, sustaining optimal levels of vitamin E and antioxidants promotes cardiovascular health as a whole.

Hydration is an additional critical element, as sufficient water consumption aids in maintaining optimal blood circulation and prevents the accumulation of blood in the vessels. Furthermore, it is advantageous to restrict sodium consumption, as an excess of salt can exacerbate symptoms associated with veins and contribute to water retention.

Although nutritional strategies offer beneficial assistance, they ought to be utilized in conjunction with professional medical advice and treatment, rather than as a substitute. Individuals who are affected by varicose veins should seek personalized guidance from healthcare professionals. In conclusion, the integration of a healthy lifestyle with a nutritionally balanced and nutrient-dense diet can make a substantial contribution to the management of varicose veins and the promotion of vascular health as a whole.

THE END

www.ingramcontent.com/pod-product-compliance
Lightning Source LLC
Chambersburg PA
CBHW070843290526
45795CB00002B/962